CONTENTS

INTRODUCTION	1
UNDERSTANDING EMOTIONS	2
The Science of Emotions	3
Identifying Your Triggers	4
The Role of Emotional Intelligence	5
TECHNIQUES FOR MANAGING EMOTIONS	7
Mindfulness and Meditation	8
Breathing Exercises	10
Cognitive Behavioral Techniques	11
DEALING WITH NEGATIVE PEOPLE	13
Setting Boundaries	14
Effective Communication	15
Empathy and Compassion	16
OVERCOMING NEGATIVITY IN THE WORKPLACE	18
Creating a Positive Work Environment	19
Handling Workplace Conflicts	21
Building Resilience	22
OVERCOMING NEGATIVITY AT HOME	24
Family Dynamics	25
Positive Parenting	26
Self-Care and Well-being	27

LONG-TERM STRATEGIES FOR EMOTIONAL MASTERY	29
Developing a Growth Mindset	30
Continuous Learning	31
Building a Support System	32
CONCLUSION	34

INTRODUCTION

In these pages, we will embark on a transformative journey—one that empowers you to understand and master your emotions, even in the face of pressure and negativity. Whether you find yourself navigating the complexities of a challenging colleague at work or the turbulence of strained relationships at home, this book offers the tools and techniques to help you manage your emotions with clarity and grace.

Emotions are at the heart of the human experience. They shape our thoughts, guide our actions, and influence every interaction we have with the world. Yet, when left unchecked, negative emotions can spiral into stress, anxiety, and even physical ailments. The good news? You have the power to change that. With the right strategies, you can reclaim control over your emotional responses, paving the way for a more positive, balanced, and fulfilling life.

In this guide, we'll explore a wide range of proven techniques—from the calming power of mindfulness and meditation to the transformative insights of cognitive-behavioral strategies. These methods will help you remain composed in adversity, and we'll also cover how to navigate negativity in others, creating a positive, resilient environment at both work and home.

By the time you reach the final page, you'll not only have a deeper understanding of your emotions but also a toolkit to manage them with confidence. Together, let's begin this journey of emotional mastery, where a brighter, more centered life awaits.

UNDERSTANDING EMOTIONS

THE SCIENCE OF EMOTIONS

Emotions are the quiet forces that shape the contours of our lives, influencing every thought, decision, and interaction. At their essence, emotions are intricate reactions that engage both the mind and body, sparked by our perceptions and deeply rooted in the brain's neural architecture—particularly in the limbic system, where the amygdala and prefrontal cortex reside.

The amygdala, often called the brain's emotional command center, is charged with detecting threats and activating our fight-or-flight response. This primal survival mechanism, though essential in ancient times, can sometimes overreact, causing heightened emotional responses to even non-threatening situations. In contrast, the prefrontal cortex acts as the brain's voice of reason, helping us regulate these impulses, allowing us to act with greater wisdom and restraint.

Understanding the neuroscience behind emotions reveals that our feelings are not random; they are the result of neural wiring and shaped by our past experiences. This knowledge arms us with the insight to begin mastering our emotions, turning them into powerful tools for positive change.

IDENTIFYING YOUR TRIGGERS

Every emotion has a source—a trigger that sparks it into being. Whether it's a fleeting thought, a painful memory, or a present-day confrontation, these triggers are pivotal in managing our emotional responses. They may be external, like a tense work environment or a disagreement with a loved one, or internal, rooted in self-doubt or unresolved past trauma.

To gain mastery over your emotions, you must first learn to identify these triggers. A simple but effective method is to keep an emotion journal. Record the situations that evoke intense emotional reactions and reflect on the underlying causes. Over time, patterns will emerge, shining a light on the specific triggers that fuel your negative emotions.

Once you understand what triggers your emotions, you can take deliberate steps to address them. This might mean adjusting your environment, challenging negative thought patterns, or seeking professional help to unpack deeper psychological issues. By gaining control over your triggers, you reduce the grip of negative emotions and pave the way for a more peaceful, balanced life.

THE ROLE OF EMOTIONAL INTELLIGENCE

Emotional intelligence (EI) is the capacity to perceive, comprehend, and regulate both your emotions and the emotions of others. It is a vital skill for successfully navigating the complexities of modern life and building meaningful connections.

EI comprises four essential pillars:

1. **Self-awareness:** The ability to recognize and understand your own emotions and their impact on your behavior and thoughts.
2. **Self-regulation:** The capacity to control impulsive reactions, manage stress, and adapt to changing circumstances with calm and poise.
3. **Social awareness:** The skill to empathize with and understand the emotions of others, attuning yourself to social dynamics and relational cues.
4. **Relationship management:** The ability to communicate effectively, resolve conflicts, and cultivate healthy, supportive relationships.

Developing emotional intelligence can transform not only your inner world but also your external reality. It equips you to handle stress with greater resilience, engage in clearer and more compassionate communication, and foster stronger, more rewarding relationships. Enhancing your EI allows you to confront life's challenges with greater ease, making you both more adaptable and emotionally grounded.

By deepening your understanding of the science of emotions, identifying your triggers, and cultivating emotional intelligence, you create the foundation for mastering your emotional landscape. This awareness is the key to unlocking a life that is not only free from the burdens of negative emotions but filled with clarity, purpose, and joy.

TECHNIQUES FOR MANAGING EMOTIONS

MINDFULNESS AND MEDITATION

Mindfulness:

Picture yourself at the edge of a tranquil lake, the water smooth as glass, mirroring the sky above without a single ripple. This is the heart of mindfulness—a state of pure awareness where you observe your thoughts and emotions without judgment. Practicing mindfulness is like training your mind to embody that calm lake, unaffected by the disturbances of stress or negativity that would otherwise ripple across your day.

When you focus fully on the present moment, you can let go of the mental noise that leads to anxiety, stress, and emotional upheaval. Scientific research strongly supports the benefits of mindfulness, showing that it significantly reduces symptoms of anxiety and depression. It also enhances self-awareness and cultivates an overall sense of well-being. By engaging in this practice, you're not just learning to cope with life's challenges but building the mental resilience to thrive in the midst of them.

Meditation:

Meditation takes mindfulness to the next level by creating a dedicated space for inner peace. Imagine sitting quietly in a peaceful room, your eyes gently closed, your breath flowing naturally. In that space, the worries and distractions that so often clutter your mind begin to dissipate, leaving room for clarity and calm.

Regular meditation rewires the brain, helping to reduce negative thought patterns, strengthen concentration, and enhance emotional stability. Studies show that meditating even for just a few minutes daily can lower stress levels, improve emotional health, and boost focus. It's a powerful tool that, over time, will transform the way you handle life's pressures, allowing you to respond with greater poise and less reactivity.

BREATHING EXERCISES

Deep Breathing:

Breathing is something we do without thought, yet it holds the key to managing stress and emotions effectively. When we engage in deep, diaphragmatic breathing, we activate our body's relaxation response, counteracting stress hormones and inducing a sense of calm. Imagine inhaling deeply, your lungs filling up with air, your abdomen expanding. As you exhale slowly, tension leaves your body with each breath.

Practicing deep breathing for just a few minutes can have immediate effects on your mood, lowering blood pressure, calming the nervous system, and restoring emotional balance. This simple technique can be practiced anytime—whether you're facing a stressful meeting at work or trying to center yourself at the end of a chaotic day.

COGNITIVE BEHAVIORAL TECHNIQUES

Cognitive Restructuring:

The thoughts we allow ourselves to dwell on shape our reality. Cognitive restructuring is a powerful technique designed to identify and challenge negative, distorted thought patterns, replacing them with healthier, more constructive ones. Imagine your mind as a garden, where negative thoughts are weeds that need to be pulled out. By practicing cognitive restructuring, you're planting seeds of positivity and nurturing a healthier mental landscape.

This technique has been highly effective in treating anxiety, depression, and other mental health challenges, providing people with a concrete way to shift their mindset. Over time, it helps you develop a more balanced, positive outlook on life, even when faced with difficult circumstances.

Thought Stopping:

Sometimes, negative thoughts can spiral out of control, leading to heightened anxiety or despair. Thought stopping is a practical tool that interrupts this cycle. Imagine a stop sign flashing in your mind when a negative thought begins to take over, reminding you to pause and replace that thought with something more positive. This technique can help you regain control over your thought processes, halting the cascade of negativity before it escalates.

By practicing thought stopping, you become more mindful of when and how negative thoughts arise, and you can break their hold before they affect your emotions and actions. It's a method that allows you to consciously choose optimism over pessimism, gradually fostering a more resilient and positive mental framework.

By incorporating mindfulness, meditation, deep breathing, and cognitive behavioral techniques into your daily life, you'll develop the tools to master your emotions. These practices empower you to navigate stressful situations, whether in the workplace or at home, with greater ease and emotional strength. Remember, the journey to emotional mastery is an ongoing process. Each technique you adopt will bring you closer to a life filled with balance, calm, and fulfillment.

DEALING WITH NEGATIVE PEOPLE

SETTING BOUNDARIES

Assertiveness Training:

Imagine standing at the edge of a wide, open field, with the space to move freely and breathe deeply. This sense of openness and security is what setting boundaries can feel like—creating a protective space where you can exist without the intrusion of others 'negativity. Establishing boundaries is not about building walls but about defining clear, respectful limits. Assertiveness training is the key to this process. It teaches you how to communicate your needs with clarity and confidence, ensuring your voice is heard without aggression or passivity.

Picture yourself in a conversation, calmly and firmly expressing your limits, much like a lighthouse standing tall amidst a storm. Assertiveness is about holding your ground with dignity and self-respect, and it not only safeguards your emotional well-being but also fosters healthier relationships. By learning to say "no" when necessary and articulating your needs, you create an environment of mutual respect and understanding in both personal and professional settings.

EFFECTIVE COMMUNICATION

Nonviolent Communication:

Words have immense power—they can heal or harm, build bridges or erect walls. Nonviolent Communication (NVC) offers an approach that transforms how we express ourselves. NVC focuses on conveying our feelings and needs without blaming or criticizing, allowing for healthier and more compassionate dialogue. Imagine a conversation where, instead of reacting with defensiveness or frustration, you speak with clarity and empathy. This approach creates a heart-centered connection, helping you navigate potentially tense situations with grace.

Practicing NVC is like speaking the language of empathy, where understanding takes precedence over judgment, and curiosity replaces conflict. By articulating your needs in a calm, non-confrontational way, you can defuse tension and transform difficult conversations into opportunities for connection. Whether at work or at home, this technique fosters a more harmonious environment and deepens your relationships.

EMPATHY AND COMPASSION

Empathy Exercises:

Empathy is the ability to step outside of yourself and into another person's world—to see through their eyes and feel with their heart. It's as if you're opening a window into someone else's inner experience, allowing you to understand their emotions and perspectives on a deeper level. Empathy doesn't just soften your interactions with others; it also reduces your own negative reactions, making you more resilient to external stressors.

Engaging in empathy exercises sharpens this skill. Picture yourself sitting with a friend who's sharing their troubles. Instead of simply hearing their words, you focus on truly feeling what they're going through. This kind of active, heartfelt listening creates a space for understanding and compassion, dissolving any negativity that might have otherwise escalated. Practicing empathy enriches not only your relationships but your emotional life as well, giving you greater insight and resilience.

By mastering these techniques—assertiveness training, effective communication, and empathy—you can navigate challenging interactions with negative people in a way that protects your emotional health. These skills empower you to set healthy boundaries, communicate effectively, and cultivate empathy, transforming potentially draining encounters into opportunities for personal growth and deeper connection.

The beauty of these practices is that they are not about changing others; rather, they are about changing how you respond to them. By mastering your own emotions and interactions, you create a more positive, fulfilling life, regardless of the negativity around you.

OVERCOMING NEGATIVITY IN THE WORKPLACE

CREATING A POSITIVE WORK ENVIRONMENT

Gratitude Practices:

Imagine walking into a workspace where appreciation flows naturally, lifting everyone's spirits as effortlessly as a fresh cup of coffee. Gratitude is a simple yet powerful force that can transform the energy of a workplace. When leaders and employees alike express gratitude regularly—whether through a verbal thank you, a written note, or a formal recognition program—it creates a ripple effect that elevates morale and fosters a culture of positivity.

Research has shown that gratitude doesn't just boost individual well-being; it also enhances team cohesion and job satisfaction. A simple habit, like starting meetings with a moment of appreciation, can shift the mood from stress-driven to purpose-driven. When employees feel seen and valued, they're more motivated and engaged, and negativity loses its grip. By incorporating gratitude practices into daily work life, you cultivate an environment where everyone feels acknowledged and eager to contribute their best.

Positive Reinforcement:

Positive reinforcement is like nourishing a garden—by acknowledging and rewarding positive behavior, you encourage growth and productivity. In a workplace setting, positive reinforcement involves recognizing employees 'efforts and achievements in ways that make them feel appreciated and inspired. This can range from informal gestures like praise during a team meeting to more formal rewards such as bonuses or awards.

When employees know their hard work is recognized, it boosts morale and keeps them engaged. Studies have shown that regular, sincere recognition enhances job satisfaction and decreases turnover. Imagine a workplace where employees are not only meeting expectations but exceeding them because they feel supported and celebrated. By cultivating a culture of positive reinforcement, you create a thriving, motivated team that's resilient in the face of challenges.

HANDLING WORKPLACE CONFLICTS

Conflict Resolution Training:

In any workplace, conflict is inevitable, but its impact depends on how it's managed. Conflict resolution training equips employees with the skills to address disagreements in a constructive, respectful way. Instead of avoiding or escalating conflicts, employees learn techniques like active listening, empathy, and problem-solving.

Imagine a workplace where conflicts are seen not as threats but as opportunities for growth and understanding. By fostering open communication and mutual respect, you can transform moments of tension into collaborative solutions, improving team cohesion and reducing negativity. Conflict resolution training ensures that issues are handled promptly and professionally, preventing simmering tensions from boiling over and creating an emotionally safe and harmonious environment.

BUILDING RESILIENCE

Resilience Training:

In the fast-paced, high-pressure environment of modern workplaces, resilience is essential for both individual and organizational success. Resilience training teaches employees how to adapt to challenges, manage stress, and bounce back from setbacks with a renewed sense of purpose. It often involves cognitive-behavioral strategies to help employees reframe negative situations and maintain a positive outlook, as well as stress-management techniques like mindfulness, physical activity, and time management.

A workforce equipped with resilience can weather challenges with grace, turning obstacles into opportunities for growth. Imagine a team that approaches each setback not with frustration, but with problem-solving and optimism. By investing in resilience training, you create a work culture where employees are mentally tough, emotionally balanced, and capable of handling adversity with poise. This, in turn, creates a healthier, more positive work environment where stress is managed effectively, and productivity flourishes.

By embracing these strategies—gratitude practices, positive reinforcement, conflict resolution, and resilience training—you can create a workplace that not only navigates negativity but thrives in the face of it. A positive work environment is not simply the absence of conflict or stress; it's a place where employees feel valued, supported, and empowered to be their best selves. When people flourish, so does the organization. This is the foundation for long-term success and a culture that both attracts and retains top talent.

OVERCOMING NEGATIVITY AT HOME

FAMILY DYNAMICS

Family Therapy:

Imagine a family sitting in a cozy, inviting room, guided by a therapist who gently helps them untangle their conflicts and improve communication. Family therapy offers a safe and structured environment for each family member to express their feelings, uncover misunderstandings, and build empathy. The therapist facilitates conversations that may be difficult to have on their own, ensuring everyone feels heard and validated. This process helps families learn healthier ways to interact, resolve disputes, and support each other.

Family therapy is particularly effective for addressing deeper, underlying issues that may be fueling negativity or tension in the household. Whether dealing with a major life event, a long-standing conflict, or everyday challenges, therapy can transform a troubled household into one of harmony, understanding, and mutual respect. The result is a stronger, more resilient family bond, where each member feels secure and supported.

POSITIVE PARENTING

Emotion Coaching:

Picture a parent kneeling down to their child's level, speaking calmly, and helping them navigate a difficult emotion like frustration or sadness. This is the essence of emotion coaching, a parenting technique that encourages children to understand and manage their emotions effectively. Instead of dismissing or punishing a child's emotional outbursts, emotion coaching acknowledges the child's feelings, helps label them, and provides guidance on how to respond appropriately.

Parents who practice emotion coaching foster emotional intelligence in their children, which research shows is crucial for building resilience and forming healthy relationships. Children learn that it's okay to have difficult emotions but that they can be managed in a constructive way. Over time, this approach reduces negativity and creates a more empathetic and supportive home environment. Emotion-coached children are better prepared to handle life's stresses and challenges with confidence and calm.

SELF-CARE AND WELL-BEING

Self-Care Routines:

Imagine starting your day with a routine that is dedicated solely to your well-being—whether it's through meditation, exercise, or simply enjoying a quiet moment with a cup of tea. Self-care is not a luxury but a necessity, especially for those juggling the pressures of family life and work. Regular self-care practices help reduce stress, increase emotional resilience, and promote a positive mindset, which in turn creates a healthier home environment.

When you prioritize self-care, you're not only taking care of yourself but also setting a powerful example for your family. Whether it's through engaging in a hobby, practicing mindfulness, or spending time in nature, self-care routines recharge your mental and physical energy, enabling you to show up as your best self. This ripple effect of well-being benefits everyone in the household, fostering a more balanced and peaceful family life. A parent or partner who practices self-care is more patient, empathetic, and better equipped to handle everyday challenges.

By focusing on these key areas—family dynamics, positive parenting through emotion coaching, and self-care—you can significantly reduce negativity at home. Family therapy can open channels of communication and resolve long-standing issues, while positive parenting helps children develop emotional intelligence. Finally, self-care ensures that you are emotionally balanced and capable of creating a nurturing, supportive atmosphere. Together, these practices lay the foundation for a harmonious, positive, and thriving home life.

LONG-TERM STRATEGIES FOR EMOTIONAL MASTERY

DEVELOPING A GROWTH MINDSET

Growth Mindset Training:

Imagine approaching every challenge with the mindset that it is a stepping stone, not a stumbling block. This is the heart of a growth mindset—the belief that abilities and intelligence are not fixed, but can be developed through effort, persistence, and learning. When you embrace challenges as opportunities for growth, you become more resilient and motivated.

Picture yourself facing a difficult project at work or attempting to learn a new skill. Instead of feeling defeated or overwhelmed, you view it as a chance to expand your capabilities. Growth mindset training teaches you to celebrate effort over perfection, to welcome constructive feedback, and to see failures as valuable learning experiences. By adopting this mindset, you begin to transform setbacks into progress, viewing obstacles as the perfect environment for growth. Over time, this shift in thinking not only enhances your emotional well-being but also strengthens your ability to maintain a positive outlook, no matter the circumstances.

CONTINUOUS LEARNING

Lifelong Learning:

Imagine yourself on a journey where every step is an opportunity to gain new knowledge, skills, and insights. This is the essence of lifelong learning—an ongoing commitment to personal and professional growth. The practice of continuous learning keeps you adaptable, curious, and motivated in an ever-changing world. Whether you're reading a new book, attending a course, or learning a new hobby, each moment of learning enriches your mind and spirit.

Engaging in lifelong learning allows you to remain open to new perspectives and to sharpen your problem-solving skills. It fosters resilience by equipping you with the tools to handle uncertainty and change. By making continuous learning a habit, you build a foundation for personal fulfillment and emotional mastery. In this way, the journey itself becomes a source of motivation, as every new lesson enhances your confidence and ability to navigate life's challenges with a positive mindset.

BUILDING A SUPPORT SYSTEM

Support Groups:

Imagine being part of a community where your struggles are understood, your experiences are validated, and your victories are celebrated. Building a strong support system, whether through formal support groups or informal networks of friends and family, is a vital aspect of emotional resilience. Support groups provide a safe space for you to share your challenges, receive feedback, and gain insight from others who are going through similar experiences.

Picture yourself attending a support group or connecting with others who share similar challenges—be it in managing stress, dealing with negativity, or coping with personal struggles. In these spaces, the collective wisdom and shared experiences of the group empower you to build emotional strength and find practical solutions to your difficulties. Support systems create a buffer against negativity by offering encouragement, understanding, and practical advice. They help you feel less isolated and more equipped to face adversity with confidence and optimism.

By cultivating a **growth mindset**, committing to **lifelong learning**, and **building a support system**, you create a solid foundation for emotional mastery. These strategies not only foster personal development but also help you stay resilient and positive in the face of adversity. Remember, emotional mastery is a journey—each step you take towards growth, learning, and connection brings you closer to a more empowered and fulfilling life.

CONCLUSION

Mastering your emotions is not a destination but a lifelong journey—one of growth, self-discovery, and transformation. The strategies laid out in this book are designed to empower you with the tools to navigate the complexities of life with grace and resilience. When you embrace these techniques, you don't just manage your emotional landscape—you reshape it. Challenges become stepping stones, and negativity turns into the catalyst for your personal evolution.

The power to craft your emotional well-being rests within you. Every step you take toward understanding and mastering your emotions brings you closer to a life that is balanced, fulfilling, and rich in purpose. Whether you're facing stress at work, conflicts at home, or the weight of personal challenges, you have the capacity not only to rise above but to truly thrive.

As you embark on this journey, remember to be patient with yourself. Change doesn't happen overnight, but every small effort you make adds to your overall progress. Celebrate your victories —no matter how small—and learn from your setbacks. Continue to cultivate a mindset of growth, persistence, and resilience. With dedication and practice, you can master your emotions, creating a life filled with positivity, joy, and meaning.

Words of Hope

In moments of uncertainty, remind yourself that you are never alone. Many have walked this path before you, emerging stronger, wiser, and more resilient. Every challenge you face is not a barrier but an invitation—an opportunity to grow, to learn, and to become a better version of yourself. Hold on to hope, for it is the beacon that will guide you through the darkest of times.

Success Stories

Consider Sarah, a young professional once paralyzed by anxiety and self-doubt in her high-pressure career. By practicing mindfulness and cognitive restructuring, she redefined her relationship with stress, transforming it into an ally rather than an enemy. Not only did Sarah excel in her work, but she also found a deeper sense of peace and confidence that permeated every aspect of her life.

Or take John, a father who struggled with constant conflict at home. Through family therapy and emotion coaching, John learned to communicate with empathy and patience, rebuilding the bonds with his children and partner. The shift in his family dynamics was nothing short of transformative, turning discord into a home filled with understanding and love.

These stories are living proof of the power of emotional mastery. They remind us that with the right mindset and the right tools, we can overcome negativity and create lives that radiate hope and possibility.

Your Journey

Your journey toward mastering your emotions is a testament to your strength, courage, and determination. Embrace this path with your whole heart, and let your growing emotional intelligence be your compass toward a future filled with harmony and fulfillment. The road ahead may not always be easy, but the rewards are profound and immeasurable. Keep moving forward, knowing that success is not just possible—it is inevitable.

www.ingramcontent.com/pod-product-compliance
Lightning Source LLC
Chambersburg PA
CBHW031514210526
45464CB00007B/2907